Diseases of the Horse's Foot

H. Caulton (Harry Caulton) Reeks

Curated Edition

Edited by David Nguyen

Edited by David Nguyen.

Contents

Synopsis

"DISEASES of the Horse's Foot" by H. Caulton Reeks is a scientific publication likely written in the early 20th century. This work focuses on the various ailments affecting horses' hooves, a crucial aspect for veterinarians and horse owners alike given the horse's dependence on sound feet for mobility and labor. The text aims to provide a comprehensive resource based on both the author's knowledge and the contributions of others, encompassing a range of anatomical and pathological studies. The opening of the text outlines the significance of understanding foot diseases in veterinary surgery, addressing common issues faced in horses, from neglected foot care in young colts to injuries sustained in different environments and the consequences of improper shoeing. It emphasizes the hoof's fundamental role in the horse's overall health and usefulness, laying a foundation for the subsequent chapters that delve into regional anatomy, physiology, and specific diseases. The author reveals that many complications can arise from insufficient knowledge in shoeing practices and stresses the importance of vigilant foot management to prevent various foot disorders.

CHAPTER XI

DISEASES OF THE BONES

. PERIOSTITIS AND OSTITIS.

We head this section, Periostitis *and* Ostitis, for the reason that in actual practice it is rare for one of these affections to occur without the other. The periosteum and the bone are so intimately connected that it is difficult to conceive of disease of the one failing to communicate itself in some degree to the other. Pathologically, however, and for purposes of description, it is more convenient to describe separately the abnormal changes occurring in these two tissues.

With the main phenomena of inflammation occurring elsewhere we presume our readers are aware. Briefly we may put it, that under the action of an irritant, either actual injury, chemical action, or septic infection, the healthy tissues around react in order to effect repair of the parts destroyed. Also that this reaction involves the distribution of a greater blood-supply to the part, with an abundant migration of leucocytes, and the outpouring of an inflammatory exudate, together with symptoms of heat, pain, redness, and swelling of the affected area. And that in chronic inflammations, owing to persistence of the cause, the process of repair thus instituted does not stop at mere restoration of lost tissue, but continues to the extent of forming an abnormal quantity of such tissue as normally exists in the parts implicated.

The process of inflammation in bone is essentially the same. It takes place along the course of the bloodvessels, and is only modified in its attendant phenomena by the structure of the parts involved. Swelling, for instance, cannot take place in the centre of compact bone tissue. Otherwise, other changes occur exactly as in inflammations of other structures.

When the causal irritant has been excessively severe and the migration of leucocytes abundant, actual formation of pus may occur, the bony tissue being broken down and mingled with it, and an abscess cavity formed. In milder cases, affected and necrotic tissue is removed by a process of phagocytosis, and new tissue (this time osseous) formed in its place.

In the periosteum we may take it roughly that inflammation runs a course similar to that occurring in soft tissues elsewhere. There is but one exception, and that, as we shall mention shortly, is connected with its deeper layer.

As we know, the periosteum consists of two layers, an outer fibrous and an inner yellow elastic, and is extremely vascular. Numerous bloodvessels ramify in it, and, with their attendant nerves, break up to enter the numberless canals of the Haversian system. This extreme vascularity, of course, favours abundant exudation. The exudate, however, is, as it were, shut in by the dense fibrous layer of the membrane, and the result is that in periostitis it collects between the membrane and the bone, causing swelling and raising of the membrane, and giving rise to excruciating pain from pressure upon the nerves.

Should the periostitis be complicated by the formation of pus, then the vessels entering and supplying the bone are, in the suppurative area, destroyed. With their destruction it may happen that we get also death of a portion of the osseous tissue. This, however, when the suppuration is abundant, cannot commonly occur, as the bloodvessels within the bone–those of the medulla–commence to supply blood to the affected part. In cases of trouble with the bones of the foot, these last few remarks have a special significance. Here we have three bones whose medullary cavity is extremely small–almost nil, in fact–which explains in some measure how easy it is when suppuration exists to get necrosis and exfoliation of, say, portions of the os pedis. Necrosis and sloughing of the periosteum itself may also happen, but as the extreme vascularity of the membrane is a fairly strong safeguard against that it is of only rare occurrence.

In connection with the deep layer of the periosteum, and forming part of it, are found numerous bone-forming cells (*osteoblasts*). These, under ordinary conditions, are relatively quiescent. Under the slightest irritation or stimulation, however, their bone-forming functions are stirred into abnormal activity, thus explaining how easy it is (especially with bones so open to receive slight injuries as are those of the foot) to get ossific deposits, the starting-point of which we are quite unable to account for

With this brief introduction we will now describe such pathological changes as occur in the separate structures, and which we are likely to encounter in the various diseases of the foot. While so doing, we shall draw attention to such diseases as we have previously described in which the pathological conditions we are considering may be met with.

1. PERIOSTITIS.

This we shall consider under *(a)* Simple Acute Periostitis, *(b)* Suppurative Periostitis, *(c)* Osteoplastic Periostitis.

(a) Simple Acute Periostitis.–This is the periostitis that follows on the infliction of a slight injury to the membrane–an injury without an actual wound and free from infective material. It is one, therefore, which we always judge as existing in those cases where we have distinct evidence or history of injury, but in which the injury has not been severe enough to lead to fracture or to the infliction of an actual wound.

Such cases may be those of lamenesses persisting after violent blows upon the foot–cases where the animal has been kicking against the stable fittings, or where the foot has been partially passed over by the wheel of a waggon. It may be, too, that in a case of 'nail-bound' a great deal of the pain and lameness is due to a simple periostitis caused by pressure of the bulged inner-layer of horn upon the sensitive structures.

Simple acute periostitis may also occur in cases where an actual wound is in existence, but where such wound, fortunately, remains aseptic. We may thus have this condition accompanying ordinary cases of pricked foot, of treads in the anterior region of the coronet, and of accidental injuries of other kinds.

In simple acute periostitis the membrane is thicker and redder than normal, and is easily stripped from the bone. As it is pulled off it is noticed that there are numerous fibril-like processes hanging to its inner surface, and which draw out from the substance of the bone. These are simply the vessels (bloodvessels and nerves) which, loosened by the inflammatory exudate, are readily detached and drawn from the Haversian canals into which they normally run. In addition to its increased redness, the membrane has a swollen and gelatinous appearance owing to its infiltration with the inflammatory discharges. Simple acute periostitis may and often does end in resolution. On the other hand, it may end in suppuration or may become chronic. If the latter, then the osteoblasts of the innermost layer become active, and abnormal deposits of bone are the result.

(b) Suppurative Periostitis.–This condition simply indicates that the inflammation is complicated by the presence of pus organisms. It is, therefore, a common termination of the simple acute form attending the infliction of a wound. The wound becomes contaminated, and the case of simple periostitis is soon changed into the suppurative form. Once having gained entrance to the wound, the pus increases in quantity, and slowly runs between the membrane and the bone. This, however, it does not do to any large extent, showing rather a tendency to penetrate the outer fibrous layer and gain the outside of the membrane.

Suppurative periostitis is met with in foot cases, commonly in connection with punctured foot. It occurs, too, as a complication in suppurating corn, in severe tread, in complicated sand-crack, as a result of the spread of suppurative matter in acute coronitis, and in sub-horny quittor.

In ordinary cases of suppurative periostitis the pus formed is yellow in colour, creamy thick, and free from pronounced odour–the so-called 'laudable' pus of the older writers. It so happens in many cases of foot trouble, however, that putrefactive organisms gain entrance side by side with those of pus. In this case the characters of the discharge are very different. It is distinctly more fluid, is of a pink or even light chocolate colour, and extremely offensive. In these instances the pus shows a marked tendency to spread, strips the periosteum from the bone, perforates the outer layer of the membrane, and finally infiltrates the surrounding tissues.

This forms a near approach to what is known in human surgery as an *infective* periostitis, and in our subjects is nearly always met with in cases of severe prick. Its rapidly spreading character makes it always a dangerous condition, and a punctured foot exuding a discharge of this nature should always be regarded as serious. The close contiguity of the joint (it can never be *far* distant in foot cases), the spreading character of the disease, and the rapidity with which the horse succumbs to arthritis, are all factors to be taken into consideration, and to lead to a warning-note being struck when attending a case of such kind.

A further instance of infective periostitis is that met with in acute laminitis. The discharge obtained from the sole in these cases very often bears the character we have just described, and when one considers the thinness of the keratogenous membrane, one is bound to admit that changes so grave occurring in it cannot fail to spread and infect the periosteum.

(c) Osteoplastic Periostitis.–This is more particularly a chronic process, and is, as the suffix '*plastic*' indicates, associated with bone-forming changes in the membrane. It may occur as a consequence of slight but continued irritation,

often without ascertainable origin (see Case 2, p. 392), or it may be the sequel of acute disease.

In this form of periostitis the membrane is again swollen and more vascular than in health, and is also easily separable from the bone. The exposed bone is generally rough, in some cases even spicular, and the inner layer of the removed membrane is rough and gritty to the touch–characters imparted to it by numerous minute fragments of bone that have been torn away with it from the more compact osseous tissue beneath.

The results of an osteoplastic periostitis are frequently met with in the bones of the foot, and are described by veterinary writers under such headings as 'Pedal Exostoses,' 'Ossifying Ostitis,' and 'Pedal Ossification' (see Figs. 152, 153, 154, and 155). In many of these cases the disease is purely chronic, and the original cause nearly always wanting. When the foot has been subjected to laminitis of some weeks' duration, the same condition is also met with, being at the same time associated with rarefactive osteoplastic ostitis, conditions which we shall shortly describe. Cases we have examined have undoubtedly shown this condition of osteoplastic periostitis, the rarefactive and osteoplastic changes in the bone itself, met with in older cases, occurring no doubt as a result of non-expansion of the horny box. So far as we are able to ascertain, there is every reason to believe that in chronic laminitis the accompanying periostitis leads to the formation of bone, and would, if it were possible, lead to increase in the size of the os pedis. If proof were wanted of this, it is only necessary to point out the increased growth at points where resistance is nil–namely, along the upper margin of the bone (see Fig. 118). However, increase in size elsewhere is prevented by the resistance of the hoof, so that, as the bone-forming process progresses, as it inevitably *must* under the inflammatory changes going on, it is, as it were, compensated for by rarefaction or bone-absorption changes occurring simultaneously with it.

2. OSTITIS.

We shall next deal with the inflammatory changes occurring in the bones themselves, and shall consider them under (*a*): Rarefying or Rarefactive Ostitis, (*b*): Osteoplastic Ostitis, and (*c*): Caries and Necrosis.

Inflammatory changes occurring in the medulla we may pass without consideration, for in the bones of the foot the medullary cavity is so small, and the changes taking place in it of such minor importance, that we may do this without in any way seriously prejudicing our work.

(a) Rarefying or Rarefactive Ostitis.–By this term is indicated an inflammation of the bone attended by its absorption, the absorption being due to the action of certain cells, termed *osteoclasts.* This condition may be due to the pressure of tumours, may occur as the result of injury when a piece of bone is stripped of periosteum, or may be the result of an inflammation occurring in the periosteum elsewhere.

A piece of bone undergoing rarefactive ostitis is redder than normal, and the openings of the Haversian canals are distinctly increased in size. As a result a greater number of them become visible. Their increase in size is due to the inflammatory absorption of the bony tissue forming them, and in the larger of them may be seen inflammatory granulation tissue surrounding the bloodvessels. This enlargement of the Haversian canals is well seen when the bone is macerated, the whole then giving the appearance of a piece of very rough pumice-stone.

This process of rarefaction or absorption of bone tissue may be confined to quite a small portion, or it may be spread over the whole of the bone, rendering it more porous than is normal, but stopping short of complete destruction of the bone tissue (a condition which is sometimes known as inflammatory osteoporosis (see Fig. 118)). In this latter case the condition is a chronic one, and the bone tissue remaining often appears to be strengthened by a compensatory process of condensation. For an example of rarefactive ostitis as met with in cases of disease of the feet, we refer the reader to laminitis (see Fig. 118). The osteoplastic or condensing process that appears to exist simultaneously with it explains, no doubt, how it is that bones so affected do not more commonly fracture.

A further example of this process is illustrated in Fig. 133. The pressure of a tumour (in this case a keraphyllocele) has led to rarefactive changes in the bone, forming a neat indentation in the normal contour of the bone which serves to accommodate the tumour.

(b) Osteoplastic Ostitis, Osteosclerosis, or Condensation of Bone.–This, too, is essentially a chronic process. It may occur as a result of, or, as we have just shown, exist simultaneously with the condition of, diffuse rarefactive ostitis. In this case there is a formation of new bone in the connective tissue surrounding the vessels in the Haversian canals. As a consequence the bone affected is greatly increased in density, and many of the Haversian canals by this means obliterated. The end result is an increase in size of the bones in such positions as the horny box admits of it, and a peculiar ivory-like change in their consistence.

For an example of this, we again refer the reader to the changes occurring in chronic laminitis.

(c) Caries and Necrosis.–*Caries* is a word which appears to be used with a considerable amount of looseness. In addition to the meaning implied by necrosis (namely, 'death' of the part), caries is generally used to indicate that there is also a condition of rottenness, decay, and stench. It is particularly applied, in fact, when the death of the bone is slowly progressive, and is due to the inroads made upon it by putrefactive or septic matter.

Necrosis of bone may be the result of any injury, such as severe blows, or pricks and stabs. In such cases it would appear that it is loss of a portion of periosteum that is the starting-point. With death of a portion of this membrane the vascular supply to a portion of the bone is cut off, and necrosis ensues. It may also result from the extension of inflammatory affections of the structures adjoining it, as, for instance, the spread of the infective material in severe tread, or the encroaches made by pus in cases of quittor, suppurating corn, or complicated sand-crack.

When the necrosed portion of bone is small, and is free from infective properties, it is quite possible that it may, as is the case with small spots of necrosis in softer tissues, be removed by a process of absorption. It must be remembered, however, that where the necrosis has occurred as a result of septic invasion this cannot be looked for, for in every case such reparative changes are worked solely by healthy tissue. If the tissues around the necrosis are engaged in dealing with organismal invasion and the poisonous products thus poured into their working area, their state of health is so weakened that they are unable to successfully combat with the two conditions simultaneously. As a consequence, the necrotic piece of bone persists, and acts as a permanent source of irritation.

It must be remembered, too, that if the dead portion of bone–even though it be free from septic matter–is very large, that it may itself act as a continual irritant, in which case it again persists, and cannot by natural means be removed.

In our cases necrosis of bone may be met with in punctured foot, in severe cases of tread, in cases of complicated crack, and in suppurating corn. It is met with, too, in navicular disease, in the extension of irritating discharges in cases of quittor, and in cases of chronic laminitis where the solar margin of the os pedis has penetrated the sole. In this latter case the protruding portion of bone is quickly denuded of its periosteum. Its blood-supply is destroyed, and necrosis follows.

Treatment.–In simple cases of periostitis, those caused by a blow but free from an actual wound, the most beneficial treatment is the continued application of cold by means of a hose-pipe or by swabs. If by these means we are successful in holding the inflammatory phenomena in check, any large formation of new bone is prevented, and the case does well.

When the case is complicated by a wound, then antiseptic measures, such as those described in the treatment of punctured foot, will at the same time have to be practised.

It must be admitted, however, that in all but the most simple cases ordinary treatment such as this is of very little use; for with only a slight exostosis in almost any position in the foot, excessive lameness presents itself and remains. In such cases nothing is left to us but the operation of neurectomy.

When the periostitis and ostitis is the result of a wound, and is complicated by caries or necrosis of the bone, the diseased portion of bone must in every case be laid bare and removed. It so happens that the majority of cases of this kind occur in positions where the diseased bone is easily got at. The lower margin of the os pedis or portions of the wings are commonly the seat of such changes. We meet with the former in cases of pricked foot, and with the latter in severe cases of tread, or as a complication in suppurating corn or in quittor. In such cases the animal must be cast and the foot secured. The wound is then followed up, the horn if necessary removed, and the bone curetted with a Volkmann's spoon; or, if showing itself as a sequestrum, removed with a scalpel and a strong pair of forceps. Care must be taken that every particle of the diseased bone is removed, and that no part of it is left to act as an after-source of irritation. With removal of the diseased portion and a strict attention to antisepsis healing soon takes place.

Reported Cases of Periostitis and Ostitis.–1. 'Figs. 150 and 151 represent the phalangeal bones of the off fore-leg of a thoroughbred horse named Osman, who was well known as a hunt steeplechaser of considerable merit in the Midland counties some twenty years ago. I may say that this horse was under my observation pretty regularly during the whole of his career, and up to the time of his death, from ruptured aorta, when eight years old. My attention was called to him as a yearling by his owner, who told me that he sometimes fancied the colt was lame. I went over to see him, and found that he was unmistakably lame on the off fore-leg. Careful examination showed no heat or enlargement anywhere. I advised rest and the colt became pretty sound, though not quite so–in fact, he never did become quite sound, and sometimes he was very lame indeed.

'Every imaginable sort of treatment was tried short of neurectomy, without avail. The curious part of the case was that there never was much heat or any apparent change of structure, nor was "pointing" a very noticeable feature. The foot always remained a good-looking one. As the horse won a good number of races he was of some value, and was seen by a good many members of the profession, who were by no means unanimous as to the cause of lameness. The favourite theory was that it was a sequence of "split pastern." A post-mortem examination showed that there was no fracture. There was no adherence of the tendon to the navicular bone nor any ulceration. The morbid changes consisted entirely of osseous deposit as shown in the photographs. The under surface of the navicular bone was much enlarged and roughened by this bony deposit, which extended on to the os pedis, causing complete anchylosis at each extremity of the navicular. The lateral cartilages were healthy. The interesting points in connection with the case are the insidious commencement of osseous disease, its extensive development, and the entire absence of any external manifestation, through its being confined entirely within the limits of the hoof.

'It should also be noted that the animal was able to undergo a severe course of training for some years, and to gallop successfully over some of the most trying courses in England. During the whole of this time he walked and galloped apparently sound, but trotted always lame, and generally dead lame.'[A]

[Footnote A: W. E Litt, M.R.C.V.S., *Veterinary Record*, vol. viii., p. 527.]

2. 'I herewith send you photographs of three cases of the above disease, occurring in the internal surfaces of the wings of the os pedis. The photos were kindly done for me by Dr. A. Lingard, Imperial Bacteriologist to Government of India. It is a cause of many cases of obscure foot lameness in India, and frequently accounts for the numerous entries on veterinary medical history sheets under the heading "Contused Foot."

'The course of the disease is as follows: The disease makes its appearance very soon after arrival in India, the animal being admitted to hospital suffering with undoubted foot lameness, generally slight. One is soon led to suspect this disease by negative symptoms of other disease being in existence. No coronary enlargement or flinching on pressure to the coronet, no shrinkage or wiring in of the heels, neither is the characteristic pointing of navicular present. In the early stages one has false hopes of recovery by finding gradual improvement for a time by fomentation and poultices, followed by irrigation and stimulants to the coronet, and perhaps the animal is discharged from hospital, to be returned after a few days worse than ever. The disease then becomes insidious and more pronounced, the nodding of the head, even at a walk, more exaggerated, and, in fact, the animal seems afraid to put his foot to the ground, and much resembles a horse with an abscess in his foot, either from prick or picked up nail. He absolutely nurses his foot. There is a certain amount of heat always present. The disease being now well developed, pressure is caused by the ends of the navicular bone, and they become involved at their points by bony deposits. The causes of this disease I attribute, firstly, to hereditary predisposition; and, secondly the exciting cause, standing confined on board ship, where no doubt pedal congestion takes place. And perhaps some subjects start it in their marches in mobs down country in Australia. Concussion may be the cause among older horses, but the specimens photographed were taken from remounts, that had either done no work or only very gentle work, in a deeply littered riding school.

'*Treatment.*–It is obvious from the position of this disease that treatment will be of no avail in producing a cure. As already stated, the disease is insidious and progressive, and it is hopeless to expect to arrest the growths once they are started. Unnerving would no doubt remove the symptom (lameness) of the disease, but an unnerved horse is not of much good for army purposes. I therefore consider that once the disease becomes firmly established it is an unfortunate and incurable one.

'Post-mortem reveals the small nodular growths on the inner surfaces of the wings of the pedal bone, and if long established the ends of the navicular bone are also involved. Exudation and gradual growth of false material around the nodules takes place, which also serves to increase pressure.'[A]

[Footnote A: Captain L.M.Smith, A.V.D., *Veterinary Record*, vol. xi., p. 229.]

3. 'This case was brought for my opinion. The horse was lame, and walked similar to one that had had laminitis, putting the heel down first upon the ground. I ordered the patient to be destroyed. You will note the ossification of the flexor pedis at its attachment to the pedal bone. I enclose photos of the ground, also of the articular, surfaces of the bone.'[A]

[Footnote A: F.B.Jones, M.R.C.V.S., *Veterinary Record*, vol. xi., p. 230.]

B. PYRAMIDAL DISEASE, BUTTRESS FOOT, OR LOW RINGBONE.

Definition.–A condition of periostitis and ostitis in the region of the pyramidal process of the os pedis, usually preceded, but sometimes followed, by fracture of the process, and characterized by deformity of the hoof and an alteration in the normal angle of the joint.

Causes.–In the majority of cases buttress foot is brought about by fracture of the pyramidal process. Thus, although distinct evidence of such is nearly always wanting, we may assume that the original cause is violent injury to the part in question. Properly, therefore, one would say that this condition should be described under Fractures of the Os Pedis. It appears, however, that other cases of the kind arise in which fracture is altogether absent, or in which it is plainly seen to be subsequent to the diseased processes in the bone. For that reason, and also for the reason that the condition has come to be known by the name we have given, we give it special mention.

Symptoms and Diagnosis.–Even when the condition arises as the result of fracture, the ordinary manifestations of such a lesion are absent. By reason of the situation of the parts within the hoof we are unable to detect crepitation, and the resulting lameness is perhaps–in fact, nearly always is–neglected until such time as any heat or swelling caused by the injury has disappeared, in which case we are denied what evidence we might have obtained from that. All that is presented is lameness, and lameness that is at times excessive. But with the lameness there is nothing distinctive. The foot is tender on percussion, and the gait suggestive of foot lameness, that is all. We are unable, therefore, to make an exact diagnosis, and the condition goes for some time undetected.

Later, however, changes in the form of the hoof and the coronet begin to appear. The skin of the coronet, especially in the region of the toe, becomes more or less thickened and indurated, and the same remark applies to the subcutaneous tissues. The most marked change, however, is the alteration in the shape of the hoof. The wall protrudes at the toe in a manner that has been termed 'buttress-like,' and has given to the condition one of its names. This, of course, entirely alters the contour of the horny box. From being more or less U-shaped, it approaches nearer the formation of the letter V, the point of the V being at the toe.

In the later stages the coronary enlargement is plainly seen to be due to an extensive formation of bone. It is, in fact, a reparative callus, and the reason it reaches so large a size is probably to be accounted for by the pull of the extensor pedis upon the detached pyramidal process. As might be expected, this displacement of the fractured portion, with its effect of giving greater length to the extensor pedis, leads to a backward displacement of the os coronæ upon the pedal bone. As a result there is a marked depression at the coronet, the depression being heightened in effect by the exostosis in front. Pyramidal disease is, as a rule, met with in the hind-feet, but occurs also in the fore.

Pathological Anatomy.–When occurring without fracture, the first observable change is a thinning of the articular cartilage of the pyramidal process, through which the bone beneath appears abnormally white. Later the thinning of the cartilage progresses until at last it becomes entirely obliterated. This destruction of the cartilage commences first at the highest point of the articular surface of the pyramid, and gradually reaches further backward into the joint. While this is taking place the new bone is being formed on the front of the os pedis, below and around the process, until, as we have already seen, an exostosis is formed, large enough to be noticeable at the coronet. This, of course, partly implicates the joint and the points of the insertion of the extensor tendon.

Finally, fracture may, or may not, take place. When it does, the exostosis is larger, and the general deformity of the hoof greater.

Treatment.–Ordinary treatment, such as point or line firing, repeated blisters, or hoof section, each of which we have tried, appears to be utterly useless. So far as we have been able to gather from the writings of other practitioners, however, neurectomy returns the animal for a time to usefulness. If the fore-limb is the seat of trouble, either plantar or median neurectomy may be practised; if the hind, then the best results are obtained by section of the posterior tibial.

Reported Cases.–1. This animal, a mare, had been rested for lameness behind for two or three weeks, and then sent out to work, going sound. This was repeated several times, and each time the coachman reported, "Goes very lame behind after she has been at work about fifteen to twenty minutes." She always pulled out sound when I saw her in a halter on the following day, so I had her ridden, and after about seven or eight minutes she began to go lame in a hind-limb. Her lameness got rapidly worse as she was being ridden, and within a quarter of mile of her first showing lameness, she dropped and carried the lame foot in a way that suggested a badly fractured pastern. There was no recognisable disease in the limb to account for this lameness.

'I divided the posterior tibial nerve, and she went back to work moving sound, and continued to work sound up to her death from one of the regularly fatal bowel lesions twist or rupture.

'She worked nearly two years after unnerving, and developed the usual thickening at the coronet.'[A]

[Footnote A: W. Willis, M.K.C.V.S., *Journal of Comparative Pathology and*

Therapeutics, vol. xv., p. 366.]

2. 'The subject of this note was a chestnut mare, nine years old, and used for omnibus work.

'*History*.–For about two months the mare was lame on the off fore-leg, and in spite of treatment the condition became steadily worse. The off fore-foot was rather long and narrow, and the fetlock-joint was inclined to be bowed outwards, but the degree of lameness was out of proportion to these defects, and the diagnosis was obscure.

'Median neurectomy was performed on May 10, 1902, and reduced the lameness to about half of what it was before. On June 5 ulnar neurectomy was performed, with the result that the mare became sound, and went to work three weeks later. She continued to work soundly and well, being inspected from time to time.

'During February of 1903 the coronet began to enlarge in front and slightly to the outer side, and gradually a ridge of bone grew down from the coronet to the toe. The case, in fact, became a typical one of so-called "buttress foot," which my friend Mr. Willis has described as diagnostic of disease of the pyramidal process of the pedal bone. Meanwhile the swelling of the coronet, which appeared to be mainly composed of fibrous tissue, increased in size, until the whole of the front and sides became involved, assuming the appearance shown in Fig. 156.

'In spite of the coronary enlargement the mare worked well, and remained free from lameness till June 8, 1903, on which day the limb became swollen up to the site of the median operation. The appearance of the limb closely simulated an attack of lymphangitis. The mare was kept under observation till the 13th of the same month, during which time the swelling increased, as did also the lameness to a slight degree. During progression she brought the heel to the ground and "rocked the toe," as in a case of rupture of the perforans tendon. The mare was killed on June 13.

'*Post-mortem.*–In trying to pull away the hoof from the sensitive structures with a pair of farrier's pincers, the tendons and ligaments of the corono-pedal articulation gave way, leaving the pedal bone *in situ.* The flexor perforans tendon showed inflammatory softening, and was very nearly ruptured through at the level of the navicular bone. There was slight evidence of navicular disease. The articular cartilage of the corono-pedal joint had been almost completely removed, and there was sclerosis of the opposed bony surfaces, which by unequal wear had brought about deformity of the os coronæ and os pedis.

There was very old-standing fracture of the pyramidal process (see Fig. 157), with the formation of a false joint between the process and the pedal bone. There was also a recent fracture of the part of the pedal bone which carries the articulation for the navicular bone, and this and the tendon lesions probably accounted for the final symptoms of 'break-down.'

Neurectomy enabled us to get a year's useful work out of what would otherwise have been a hopeless cripple.[A]

[Footnote A: A.R. Routledge, M.R.C.V.S., *Journal of Comparative Pathology and Therapeutics*, vol. xvi., p. 371.]

C. FRACTURES OF THE BONES.

More or less by reason of the protection afforded them by the hoof fractures of the bones of the foot are rare. When occurring they are more often than not the result of direct injury, as, for example, violent blows, the trapping of the foot in railway points, the running over of the foot with a heavily-laden waggon, or violent kicking against a gate or a wall. They occur also as a result of an uneven step upon a loose stone when going at a fast pace, and as a result of sudden slips and turns, in which latter case they are met with when animals have been galloping unrestrained in a field, or when an animal, ridden or driven at a fast pace, is suddenly pulled up, or just as suddenly turned.

At other times fractures in this region take place without ascertainable cause, and cases are on record where animals turned overnight into a loose box in their usual sound condition have been found in the morning excessively lame, and fracture afterwards diagnosed.

1. FRACTURES OF THE OS CORONÆ.

Fractures of the os coronæ result from such causes as we have just enumerated, and are nearly always seen in conjunction with fractured os suffraginis. When this latter bone is also fractured diagnosis is comparatively easy, a certain amount of crepitus, even when the suffraginis is only split, being obtainable. When the os corona alone is fractured then diagnosis is extremely difficult, the smallness of the bone and the comparative rigidity of the parts rendering manipulation almost useless, and effectually preventing the obtaining of crepitus. It is, in fact, only when the bone is broken into many pieces that crepitus may be detected, and even then it is slight.

Reported Cases.–1. 'The subject was a four-year old hunter. While at exercise in the morning of August 10 he bolted, got rid of his rider, and ran about in a mad fashion, came into contact with a wheelbarrow in a narrow passage, and finally came into violent contact with a wall, which had the effect of throwing him down. The rider stated that the animal suddenly put down his head and managed to get off the bridle; he then bolted, and the only chance for the rider was to throw himself off.

'On examination I found the horse unable to place any weight on the off fore-leg, the pastern was swollen and painful, the hollow of the heel was also swollen, and there was marked constitutional disturbance.

'After a short time he would place the heel on the ground and elevate the toe to a slight degree. On manipulating the pastern slight crepitation could be discovered, and there was abnormal mobility in the corono-pedal articulation. On the near fore-leg there were extensive wounds in the region of the knee, and great laceration of the tissues. The animal was destroyed.

'On examining the leg I found the subcutaneous tissues infiltrated from below the knee to the foot, large masses of gelatinous blood-stained material being present along the flexor tendons and in the hollow of the heel. The inferior articular surface of the os suffraginis was denuded of cartilage anteriorly; the os coronæ was fractured into eight moderate sized, irregular fragments, and ten minute pieces. The surface of the perforans tendon as it glides over the smooth surface at the back of the os coronæ was lacerated, and minute portions of the bone were found embedded therein.'[A]

[Footnote A: E. Wallis Hoare, F.R.C.V.S., *Veterinary Record*, vol. xiv., p. 133.]

2. 'Here, again, fracture was the result of the animal bolting with his rider. Trying to avoid collision with a conveyance coming towards him, the animal slipped on a wooden pavement, sliding along until his near fore-leg came in contact with the wheel of a standing cab. There was considerable swelling from the knee downwards, great pain, and evidence of fracture in the region of the pastern.

'Post-mortem revealed the os suffraginis broken into about thirty pieces, and the os coronæ with a piece broken off the inside of its proximal end.[A]

[Footnote A: A.F. Appleton, M.R.C.V.S., *Veterinary Journal*, vol. xiii., p. 411.]

3. 'The patient was a brown mare used for heavy van work in London. About January 10 she was lame, and as she had a cracked heel, was treated by poulticing for a day, and then by antiseptic lotions. In a week she was sent to work, but the following day lameness returned, and continued till about February 15. No special symptom was detected which indicated the exact position of any cause of lameness. Then the lameness increased in severity, and some swelling around the coronet began to show itself.

'In consultation with another veterinary surgeon, two possible causes of this intense lameness were discussed: one, that we had septic infection of the coronet, and that probably the swelling of this part would soften, and sloughs occur; the other, that a fracture of the os pedis or os coronæ existed. The enlargement of the coronet was hard and firm, not particularly sensitive. It was decided to do nothing for a few days. In a week the pain abated, and the mare would put her foot on the ground, and ceased to "nurse" the limb as she had done. When moved over in the box she put a little weight on the foot, but limped very decidedly.

'Another week passed, and the pain and lameness further abated, but the swelling around the coronet continued. Perhaps it was a little less in front, but it had not decreased on the inside. It remained firm, and was not painful on pressure. It showed no soft places, and the upper part of the leg remained free from oedema.

'The diagnosis was now that a fracture existed, and it was proposed to send the mare to grass for a few months. The consulting veterinary surgeon suggested that before doing so a blister might be applied to the coronet. This was done. The mare was found next day again on three legs. She had apparently been down during the night. In a few days the coronet increased again in size, and within a week "broke out" in two places.

'The opinion now formed was that, with a fracture and this additional cause of inflammation around the joint, it would be most economical for the owner to have her killed. This was done, and a post-mortem examination was made by Mr. Hunting and Mr. Willis.

'*Post-mortem.*–The foot, cut off at the fetlock-joint, showed extensive swelling all round the coronet. There were two wounds on the skin–one on the front of the coronet, the other on the inner side. From both pus and blood had escaped. They both communicated under the skin with a large abscess cavity. The abscess did not communicate with the joint. The pastern bone was sound. On separating the pastern from the coronet bone the articular surfaces were of a healthy colour, but the soft tissues immediately surrounding them were inflamed. On the centre of the articular surface of the coronary bone a thin red ring was noticed, and the portion of cartilage within it seemed raised. With the point of a scalpel this portion was lifted, and was found to be not only cartilage, but a layer of bone completely detached from the os coronæ. On removing the bones from the hoof the rest of the bone was quite normal, as was the pedal bone.

'Fig. 158 shows the articular surface of the coronet with the fracture *in situ*; and Fig. 159 the surface from which the broken portion is removed and laid to the side of the foot.

'Some interesting questions arise. How was the fracture caused? When did it occur? Between the broken portion and the main bone there was a layer of granulation tissue, so that it is certain the injury existed before the blister was applied, and it may possibly have existed from the commencement of the lameness.'[A]

[Footnote A: R. Crawford, M.R.C.V.S., *Veterinary Record*, vol. viii., p. 478.]

2. FRACTURES OF THE OS PEDIS.

These also are a result of the causes we have before given. The os pedis is also liable to fractures from pricks, from treads in the region of the wings, and from the malnutrition and careless use of the foot sometimes following neurectomy.

It is interesting to note that, with fracture of this bone, lameness is nearly always excessive, but that at times it may be entirely absent. Crepitus is, of course, denied us, and in nearly every instance the case is only diagnosed when the lameness persists and pus commences to form, or when grave changes in the normal shape of the foot compel our attention to the parts. When it is the continued formation of pus that draws our notice to something more than ordinarily grave, it is in giving exit to the pus that the fracture is nearly always discovered.

Reported Cases.–Two interesting cases of fractured os pedis are reported by Mr. Gladstone Mayall, M.R.C.V.S., in the *Veterinary Record*, vol. xiv., p. 54:

1. 'The horse was brought in markedly lame on the off hind-foot, knuckling at the fetlock, and taking a long stride with the injured limb. There was a punctured wound at the toe. The horn was pared, and antiseptic poultices applied. Notwithstanding the antiseptic treatment pus continued to form. At the end of a week sufficient horn was removed to ascertain the cause of the constant suppuration. A movable object was found at the bottom of the wound, and a piece of bone as large as a sixpence finally removed. Recovery was uneventful.'

2. 'A filly was attended for a discharging fistula at the coronet. Externally it had all the appearances of a quittor. At first no history was given. The filly went scarcely lame at all, and had never been shod. Treatment with poultices and caustic injections was useless. Finally the filly was cast and the foot examined. A piece of bone, apparently part of the wing of the os pedis, was removed, and the case made a good recovery. Subsequent inquiries elicited the fact that the animal had kicked at and hit a gate-post, and it was judged that then the injury had occurred.'

3. 'The subject was a bay horse, nine years old, used for railway shunting. On August 7 he was found to be intensely lame of the near hind-limb, and, after inquiries, there was no evidence bearing on the cause, as is often the case, and at times this comes to light when least expected.

'I was called in consultation on September 2, and found him suffering acute pain, with great swelling around the coronet. The foot was examined thoroughly, and the diagnosis was fracture of the pedal bone, and immediate slaughter was recommended. However, that was not carried out, and he died on September 22.

'The post-mortem inspection revealed a complete fracture of nearly the whole of the articulating surface and the left wing of the pedal bone (as shown in Fig. 160).'[A]

[Footnote A: J. Freeman, M.R.C.V.S., *Veterinary Journal*, vol. xxxi., p. 324.]

4. A further interesting case is reported by Mr. William Hurrell.[A] Here the cause was presumably galloping in the field, for the subject, a cart mare running out at grass with her foal, was suddenly found to be lame.

[Footnote A: *Ibid.*, vol. v., p. 408.]

As the lameness continued to increase in severity, Mr. Hurrell was called in on August 1, and diagnosed the case as one of foot lameness. On this date the foot was pared out, and a large accumulation of pus discovered, Poulticing and antiseptic dressings were continued until August 16, when a movable piece of the os pedis was found at the toe.

On August 25 this detached portion of the bone was removed, and turned out to be the whole of the anterior margin of the os pedis, measuring 3-1/2 inches long, and varying in width from 1/2 inch to 1-1/2 inches. On September 20 the mare was working without lameness.

3. FRACTURES OF THE NAVICULAR BONE.

Hidden within the wings of the os pedis, and protected as it is by its tendinous covering and the yielding substance of the plantar cushion, the navicular bone is even less liable to fracture than either of the other bones of the foot.

The most common cause of fracture of the navicular is that of stabs or deep pricks in the region of the point of the frog (see p. 216). Following that, the next most common cause is violent injury. We thus find the navicular bone fractured, together with one or both of the other bones of the foot, when the foot is run over by a heavy vehicle. One such case is reported by Mr. J.H. Carter, F.R.C.V.S., where the horse's foot was run over by a tram-engine, in which the os pedis and the navicular were fractured in several places.[A] A further case is on record where a sharp blow on the front of the hoof was the cause. In this case the os pedis and other structures were uninjured, but the navicular bone was fractured into three large, and about half a dozen small, pieces.[B]

[Footnote A: *Veterinary Journal*, vol. xxxi., p. 246.]

[Footnote B: *Veterinarian* for 1857, p. 73.]

Fractures of the navicular may occur, however, in which history of a prick or of a violent injury is absent. See reported case below.

As with fractures of the os pedis and the os coronæ, so with this exact diagnosis is difficult–we may say almost impossible. With a history of violent injury, however, some little regard may be paid to a continued heat and tenderness of the foot, and a distinct inclination on the part of the animal to go on the toe. Even when the fracture is the result of a prick, and the bone is plainly felt with the probe, we still cannot be positive as to fracture.

Reported Case.–'The animal was a Hungarian, a troop-horse in the 3rd Hussars (G. 15). On November 22, 1881, on the march from Norwich to Aldershot, the horse suddenly made a violent stumble, very nearly coming on to his knees. The rider declared that he put his foot on a stone. The accident caused great lameness in the near fore-leg, and the horse had to be led the remainder of that day's march. On the following day he was also led; but, after going some sixteen or eighteen miles, he was so lame that he was left at the nearest billet (in Edmonton). He was here attended by Mr. Stanley, M.R.C.V.S., of Edmonton, who pronounced it a case of navicular disease. I first saw the animal on December 1, 1881, and quite agreed with Mr. Stanley that it was a case of foot lameness, though, from the horse's former history, I could not think it a case of ordinary navicular disease. I diagnosed it a case of fracture, without displacement, either of the os coronæ or the navicular bone, but was more inclined to the former than the latter. This was after a full hour's examination. I failed to find any heat in, or any flinching by manipulation of, any part of the limb; but, in walking, the horse was excessively lame, going on the toe, and, indeed, trying if possible to keep the foot entirely off the ground.

'On December 6 the horse was sent on to Aldershot by rail. He was then walking better, though still very lame. My only treatment for a short time was to apply cold water constantly to the coronet and foot. For two hours daily this was done by a hose, the remainder of the time by a cold swab. On December 14 I applied a strong blister over the coronet, reaching up to the fetlock. This was washed off about the end of December. The horse was then not nearly so lame. I then resumed the cold-water treatment, and he got gradually better, and was sent to light duty on February 18, 1882. He, however, only attended one field-day, and was taken into the Horse Infirmary again on March 8, very lame. Again, there was an entire absence of heat or pain on pressure, but the same action, viz., going on the toe. I forgot to remark that he always pointed the toe of the affected leg when standing in the stable, and this symptom continued. I put him under the cold-water treatment for a short time, and about the middle of March again applied a strong blister over the coronet up to the fetlock. This was washed off about the end of the month, and was succeeded by the cold water again. Towards the end of April there was no improvement at all, and I applied for permission to destroy the horse. This was carried out on April 27, at the recommendation of Mr. Gudgin, I.V.S., Aldershot, and a Board of veterinary surgeons.

'On making the post-mortem examination I first thought the bone was only partly fractured or cracked, but on manipulating it, after its being in hot water a short time, I saw the fracture was complete.'[A]

[Footnote A: S.W. Wilson, M.R.C.V.S., A.V.D., *Veterinary Journal*, vol. xv., p. 12.]

Treatment of Fractures of the Bones of the Foot.–It will be seen at once that in most cases anything in the way of bandaging is well-nigh useless. When the os coronæ is fractured, however, a little more may be added to the natural rigidity of the parts by enclosing the region of the pastern and the foot in a plaster-of-Paris bandage. The main treatment, however, in every case, will be a continual use of the slings for at least seven to eight weeks, by that means compelling the animal to give to the injured parts the necessary amount of rest.

With fracture of the os pedis, when such is caused by pricks and complicated by a flow of pus, then attention must be given to removal of the displaced piece of bone. The pus track is to be followed up with the searcher, sufficient horn removed with the knife, and the broken piece of bone removed with a scalpel and a pair of strong forceps, the operation to be afterwards followed up by antiseptic dressings to the opening. Until this is done the wound refuses to heal.

Fracture of the navicular bone, if in any way diagnosed with certainty, offers us an almost hopeless case, for it appears to be a commonly reported fact that attempts at reunion are rare. This, in all probability, is due to the pressure put upon it every now and again, when the animal's weight presses the bone between the os coronæ and the os pedis above and the perforans tendon below. Even should reunion take place, the resulting callus, interfering as it does with the movements of the perforans, leaves us a case of incurable lameness. When the fracture is complicated by the formation of pus, as in the case of prick, then the case, with the attendant purulent synovitis and arthritis, is even more hopeless still.

Diagnosis of fracture of either of the bones of the foot is, as we have said before, extremely difficult. It so happens, therefore, in those cases caused by violent blows, that anything approaching an accurate opinion cannot be given until some months after the injury. After some time we are met with unmistakable changes in the form of the foot, and are able to assume that the persisting lameness is due to pressure of a reparative callus within the hoof. In such cases the only treatment of any use is that of neurectomy.

CHAPTER XII

DISEASES OF THE JOINTS[A]

[FOOTNOTE A: Properly speaking, we have in the foot of the horse but *one* joint–namely, the corono-pedal articulation.

Although not a joint in the strict sense of the word, we, nevertheless, intend here to consider the navicular bursa as such. In this apparatus, although we have no articular cartilage proper, and no apposition of bone to bone, we still have a large synovial cavity, and in close proximity to it bone. We may, in fact, and do get in it exactly similar changes to those termed 'synovitis' and 'arthritis' elsewhere. Therefore, we include the changes occurring in it in this chapter, and hence the plural use of the word to which this note refers.]

A. SYNOVITIS.

Definition.–By the term 'synovitis' is indicated an inflammation of the synovial membrane. It may be either (*a*) *Simple* or *Acute*, or it may be (*b*) *Purulent* or *Suppurative*.

In the simple form there is little or no tendency for the affection to implicate the other structures of the joint, whereas in the suppurative form the joint capsule, the ligaments, and the bones soon come to participate in the diseased processes, giving us a condition which we shall afterwards describe as acute arthritis.

(*a*) SIMPLE SYNOVITIS.

1. *Acute–(Causes)*.–Simple or acute synovitis is nearly always brought about by injury to the joint–by blows or bruises, or by sprains of the ligaments. At other times it occurs without ascertainable cause, and is then put down to the influence of cold, or to poisonous materials (as, for example, that of rheumatism) circulating in the blood-stream.

Pathology.–Uncomplicated acute synovitis never causes death. The pathological changes in connection with it have therefore been studied in cases purposely induced, and the animal afterwards slaughtered. It is then found that, as in inflammation elsewhere, the synovial membrane is showing the usual inflammatory phenomena–that it is thick and swollen as a result of the inflammatory hyperæmia and commencing exudation. Later, the synovial fluid becomes increased in quantity, is thin and serous, and after a time is seen to be mixed with the inflammatory exudation poured into it. We then find that it has lost its clear appearance, has become thick and muddy, and has floating in it flakes of fibrin.

If the case progresses favourably these materials are soon absorbed and resolution occurs. In rarer cases the thickening and congestion of the membrane increases, and the articular capsule becomes so distended with the increased synovia and accumulated inflammatory discharges that a kind of chemosis occurs. In other words, there oozes through, without actual rupture of the membrane, a thin, blood-stained, and purulent-looking discharge.

It is an important point to note that in cases of synovitis the fringes of the synovial membrane become swollen and blood-injected, forming noticeable red elevations at the margins of the cartilages. It is then that the diseased condition soon spreads and runs into arthritis.

Further, it is important, especially with regard to the question of the degree of pain and lameness likely to be caused, to note that often granulations are thrown out upon the looser folds of the membrane. As these increase in size they come to form fringed and villous membranous projections inserting themselves between the bones forming the articulation. In such cases there is no doubt that the intense pain sometimes observed in these cases is due to pinching of these prolongations of the synovial membrane by the opposing bones of the joint.

Symptoms and Diagnosis.–Acute synovitis of a joint leads to heat of the parts, pain, distension of the capsule, and, where the joint may be easily felt, fluctuation. In the articulation with which we are dealing, however, these last two symptoms are not easily detected, for the surrounding structures–namely, the lateral and other ligaments of the joint, the extensor pedis tendon in front, and the perforans behind, together with the dense and comparatively unyielding nature of the skin of the parts–are such as to prevent distension and fluctuation becoming marked to a visible extent. We are able to diagnose the case as one of foot lameness, and, with a history of a severe blow or other injury, are able to assume that this condition, perhaps attended with periostitis, is in existence.

When other symptoms present themselves diagnosis may be more certain. The animal becomes slightly fevered, throbbing pains in the joint manifest themselves by irregular pawing movements on the part of the patient. The animal comes out from the stable stiff, even dead-lame, and the limb is carried with the lower joints semiflexed. The breathing is hurried and the pulse firm and frequent, while in a bad case patchy perspiration breaks out at intervals on various parts of the body. If with this we get a puffy and tender swelling in the hollow of the heel, our diagnosis may be certain at any rate as to the existence of joint trouble, although, from reasons we have given, we may not be able to mark its exact nature.

2. *Chronic.*–Simple synovitis may in many instances become chronic. In this case we have simply a pouring into the synovial capsule of serous fluid, and

with it an increased quantity of synovia–this time with an absence of the usual inflammatory phenomena. Beyond the swelling of the capsule there is little to be noticed. The joint becomes perhaps a little weaker, but pain or tenderness and heat are entirely absent. Such a condition, by reason of the natural rigidity of the parts, is not to be observed in the foot, although at times it must most certainly occur. Examples of such a condition are to be found in bog-spavin, in hygroma of the stifle, and sometimes in the fetlock. From a study of these, we know that they may be induced by frequent attacks of acute synovitis, from repeated slight injuries or bruises, or from strains to the ligaments of the joint; or that they may be chronic from the outset. We know, too, that in such cases the synovial membrane becomes thickened, and that in places it may have extended somewhat over the edges of the articular cartilages. It is only fair to suppose that such changes occur also in the pedal articulation. In that case we may take it for certain that the natural rigidity of the surrounding structures has the effect of pushing the thickened membrane further between the bones of the joint than occurs in a like condition elsewhere, leading, of course, to a lameness that is marked in degree but occult as to cause.

In our minds there is no doubt that many of the occult and chronic forms of foot-lameness we meet with in practice are in this way to be accounted for. We may, in fact, explain them by suggesting either a chronic synovitis alone, or a synovitis complicated with periostitis.

Treatment of Synovitis.–If a joint has been injured, as we have suggested, by slight blows or other causes–in other words, if the injury is subcutaneous, and no wound is in existence–then there is no treatment which offers better results than does the continued application of cold.

At the same time, the animal should be slung, or, if non-excitable and inclined to rest, allowed at intervals to lie on a thick and comfortable straw bed, the cold fomentations during such intervals being discontinued. When the case is a marked one and the animal valuable, benefit will be derived from the application of crushed ice.

The animal's condition must be watched, and the case helped as far as is possible by the administration of a mild dose of physic, by saline drinks, and, when necessary, by the giving of small but repeated doses of Fleming's tincture of Aconite in order to relieve the pain. In a chronic case the repeated application of a blister is indicated.

(b) PURULENT OR SUPPURATIVE SYNOVITIS.

In this condition we have synovitis complicated by the presence of pus. Unlike the simple form, it shows a marked disposition to spread, and quickly involves the surrounding structures. Very soon the ligaments of the joint, the periosteum, the articular cartilages, and the bones are implicated. This, of course, constitutes a condition of acute purulent arthritis. Under that heading, therefore, the condition will be later discussed.

B. ARTHRITIS.

(a) SIMPLE OR SEROUS ARTHRITIS.

With an attack of simple synovitis it may be always assumed that the changes commenced in the synovial membrane, communicate themselves more or less readily to the surrounding tissues, and are not confined to the synovial membrane alone. We may thus have the inflammatory phenomena asserting themselves in the surrounding ligaments, in the periosteum, in the bone, and in the articular cartilages. It depends, in fact, upon the severity of our case whether we call it synovitis or arthritis. The two conditions merge so the one into the other that no hard-and-fast rule may be laid down whereby they may with certainty be differentiated. Such symptoms, therefore, as we have given for synovitis may be also read as indicating a condition of simple arthritis. The course of the case will be very similar, and the treatment to be followed identical with that just given.

(b) ACUTE ARTHRITIS.

Causes.–An attack of acute arthritis may commence with the affection of the synovial membrane, and spread from that to the other structures. In other cases the disease of the synovial membrane, and after it the disease of the joint, may be secondary to diseases commencing in the structures around the joint. This affection may therefore follow on a case of acute coronitis, a case of suppurating corn, a case of quittor, a severe case of tread, or may attend a case of laminitis.

Symptoms.–In our cases we get very little beyond a magnification of such symptoms as we have described under acute synovitis. The heat and the pain is perhaps greater, and the lameness more marked. It is rather to the constitutional disturbance we must look, however, for a confirmation of our opinion that arthritis is in existence. This is always severe, and of an acute febrile nature. The pulse is fast, thin, and thready, the respirations enormously increased, and the temperature high. The appetite is in abeyance, the animal quickly becomes what is termed 'tucked-up,' or greyhound-like, in the body, and patchy perspirations break out about him. The limb is held with the joints all semiflexed, and severe and intense throbbing pains are indicated by the frequent pawing movements the animal makes in the air. Manipulation of the foot is resented, and the agonizing intensity of the pain so caused is shown by the drawn and haggard appearance of the eyes.

In a favourable case the symptoms from now onwards may gradually subside. The appetite returns, the breathing and other signs of disturbance show a return to the normal, weight is placed on the limb, and resolution slowly but surely takes place. In many of these, our favourable cases, however, resolution is incomplete, and recovery only takes place at the expense of anchylosis of the joint, a condition we shall refer to later.

In unfavourable cases, and these unfortunately are only too common, the condition terminates in suppuration.

(c) PURULENT OR SUPPURATIVE ARTHRITIS.

Definition.–By this term we indicate an arthritis complicated by the formation of pus within the joint.

Causes.–The organisms of pus may infect the joint by extension of a suppurating process from without. For example, in the case of a suppurating corn, in quittor, in tread, or in the case of a suppurating wound caused by a prick, the pus formed may in many instances be very near the capsular ligament of the articulation. Under such circumstances, unless there is a free and unhindered flow of the pus from an outside opening, inroads will be made by it upon the thin capsule. The latter is quickly penetrated, and pus is admitted to the interior of the joint.

In other cases infection of the joint may proceed from within, from a poisoned state of the blood-stream. The condition occurs, for instance, in bad attacks of laminitis. We ourselves, too, have seen two cases where suppuration of the pedal articulation occurred in the septic pyæmia of foals, a disease known commonly as 'joint-ill,' and characterized by an infected state of the circulation. Cases have also come under our notice where this condition has resulted from slight injuries in the region of the insertion of the extensor pedis inflicted by the animal himself when galloping away.

Perhaps, however, the most common cause of suppurative arthritis in the foot is direct penetration of the articulation in the case of pricks. The penetrating object is nearly always dirty–bacterially dirty, at any rate–and suppuration only too readily commences. Even should such a wound be inflicted by an aseptic body, infection would quickly ensue as a result of the wound gathering dirt from the ground, or even from admission to the joint of impure and bacilli-laden air.

Symptoms and Diagnosis.–This is one of the most serious conditions we are called upon to face when dealing with diseases of the foot, for in many cases it quickly ends in exhaustion and death of the patient, while in even the most favourable cases nothing better than a condition of complete and bony anchylosis is to be expected. The owner, therefore, should be warned accordingly.

As in the other joint affections, so here, we get all the symptoms of acute febrile constitutional disturbance. The pulse, the temperature, the respirations, and the general haggard, 'tucked-up,' and distressed appearances of the animal all tell too plain a tale. Our patient is in constant pain, and the seat of the trouble is clearly enough shown by the constant pawing movements of the affected foot. If he has room to get up and down in comfort the animal adopts for long periods at a stretch the recumbent position, and is not upon his legs long enough to take the necessary amount of food to keep him going. Even when down, it is plain to see that the animal is not at rest. The pawing movement is still maintained with the foot, and every now and again the eyes are opened and the headed lifted to give a troubled look round. The appetite, too, is capricious, and in many cases almost entirely lost.

In some slight degree the condition is less to be feared in a fore than in a hind foot–that is, so far as absolutely fatal results are concerned. With the condition confined to one fore-foot, the animal is able to get up and down with a moderate degree of comfort. At intervals, therefore, he rises to take nourishment, and as soon as his wants are satisfied again lies down.

With the disease in a hind-foot matters are not taken so comfortably. The patient finds that with each day's increasing weakness the difficulty that at first he had to raise himself with only one sound hind-foot becomes enormously increased. The consequence is that he fears to go down, and the standing position is maintained until sheer weakness overcomes him, and he goes down, not to rise again without assistance.

If judiciously attended he is, of course, put in slings before this stage is reached; but there are instances, as in the case of a cart-mare heavy with foal, where the use of slings is most decidedly contra-indicated.

If doubt before existed as to the nature of the case, it is at a later stage dispelled by the appearance, generally in the hollow of the heel, of a hot and painful swelling. This at first is hard, but later fluctuates. Finally it breaks at one or more spots, and there exudes from the opening or openings a purulent and oftentimes sanious discharge, which coagulates about each fistula after the manner of ordinary synovia.

With the discharge of the abscess contents there is some slight improvement in the symptoms. Here, with a suitable treatment, and with a patient of a particularly robust constitution, the case appears to turn, and slowly but surely progresses towards the only end we can hope for–namely, a more or less painless anchylosis of the articulation.

In less favourable cases the purulent discharge continues, and (always a bad sign) becomes more or less chocolate-like in colour, distinctly thin, and stinking. The diseased process spreads until the ligaments of the joint, both by reason of their infiltration with the inflammatory discharges, and also on account of the ravages made on them by the invading pus, either greatly stretch or altogether rupture.

The joint, after its ligaments have been destroyed in this manner, is loosened, and the bones are now freely movable. Their manipulation gives to the touch a sickening, grating sound–in other words, we have crepitus. This, of course, indicates that the articular cartilages have become greatly eroded by the inflammatory process, and so left what we may term 'raw' surfaces of bone to rub together. When the animal is put to the walk the toe of the foot is elevated, and the extreme mobility of the foot gives one the idea of fracture. With every step there is a peculiar sucking noise, comparable to that of a foot moving in a boot of water, and putrescent matter is squeezed from every opening each time the foot is put to the ground. Although we have seen cases even advanced thus far recover, it is questionable whether it is now wise to attempt to prolong life. Slaughter is far more humane, and, in our opinion, except with a valuable brood animal, more economical.

If the animal is allowed to linger, other symptoms will nearly always present themselves before death occurs. Whether in slings or not, a careful watch should be kept upon the sound limb. For some time the patient stands upon it incessantly, but sooner or later it happens that a farther visit show us the animal standing with full weight on the diseased foot, and making painful pawing movements with what before was the sound. We immediately jump to the conclusion 'laminitis.' And so it is, but it is a laminitis brought about by pyæmia. This is indicated by the swollen and oedematous nature of the lymphatics of the limb. Plainly enough they indicate the road by which the poison has travelled. It is in this way: Pus and putrefactive organisms have gained entrance to the lymphatics of the original diseased limb. From these they have rapidly gained the blood-stream and set up infection elsewhere. In this particular instance it is demonstrated by the laminitis and lymphangitis of the previously sound limb. With the poison thus circulating in the blood-stream, we often also get spots of infection commenced in one or other of the more vital organs–notably the lungs or the kidneys. The end of our case is then either a gangrenous pneumonia or complications induced by a condition of widespread pyæmia.

With the animal in slings there are one or two other symptoms that call for attention. In many cases, especially with animals of a lymphatic and indolent nature, the use made of them is inordinate. The patient rests so continually in them that alarming swellings commence to make their appearance about the rectum, or in the case of a mare about the vulva. The animal must then be let down at regular intervals and again raised when rest is obtained.

A more alarming symptom still is when the animal, instead of resting in the slings by his buttocks, casts his weight bodily into the belly-rest and hangs with a heavy head into the head-stall. This indicates complete exhaustion and a wish for death. Matters should therefore be explained to the owner, and his consent obtained for immediate destruction.

Pathology.–The pathological changes occurring in suppurative arthritis we shall pass over briefly. It is almost sufficient, in fact, to say that the whole of the joint becomes completely disorganized.

The synovial membrane becomes so tremendously thickened and injected as to be scarcely recognisable as such, the thickening in the later stages being due to large growths of granulation tissue which entirely alter the appearance of the membrane as we know it normally. In the early stages the contents of the joint are composed of thin pus and synovia. Later, as destruction of the synovial membrane proceeds, the flow of synovia is stopped, while the pus formation goes on until finally nothing but pus and dead tissue products fill the cavity.

If the suppurative process has commenced from within, the pus that is formed is, as a rule, thick and creamy, comparatively unstained, and free from marked odour. If, on the other hand, air has gained access to the joint, or the suppurative process has started from the materials introduced by a foreign body, the joint contents are thin, blood-stained, and stinking.

The inflammatory changes in the joint soon spread to the ligaments, and to the soft structures in contact with them. This means that the ligaments become infiltrated with inflammatory exudate, that the fibrous bundles composing them become separated, and that the ligaments are weakened and easily stretched. As a consequence, a certain amount of displacement or dislocation of the bones is allowed.

In like manner the inflammatory changes keep spreading until we have the periosteum next the ends of the bones affected. The periostitis thus set up invariably takes the osteoplastic form, and as a result of this we have growths of new bone in the near neighbourhood of the joint. It is in the later stages of the disease–that is, when the pus has been evacuated and reparative changes commenced–that this osteoplastic periostitis is most marked, and it plays a large part in bringing about the condition of anchylosis, which we shall afterwards describe.

Grave changes also occur in the articular cartilages. They quickly lose their peculiar glistening polish, their semitransparency is lost, and the natural tint of a pearl-like blue gives way to a dirty yellow. Later this is followed by erosion of the cartilages at such points as they happen to be in greatest contact. The ends of the bones are thus exposed, and their medullary cavities exposed to infection. As a result we get in them the changes we have already described under Ostitis.

Treatment–(a) Preventive.–Seeing that many of these cases have their starting-point in stabs or penetrating wounds of the sole, we shall be concerned first with a consideration of the correct treatment to be adopted when we know the wound to have reached the articulation.

Only too frequently the treatment practised is that of poulticing. In other portions of this work we have pointed out the advantages that a continued antiseptic bathing has over the application of a poultice, the greater readiness with which the solution comes into contact with the deeper parts of the wound, and the far greater chance there is of maintaining water in an antiseptic condition than there is of keeping a poultice in the same state. There is no doubt, that in this case also, the cold or warm antiseptic bath is to be preferred to the poultice. It is questionable, however, whether even the bath is sufficient for our purpose here. We have in this case a deep punctured wound, and a wound that in every probability is infected with the organisms of pus or of putrefaction. It is a wound, moreover, which is likely to impede the thorough access to it of the solution in which the foot is fomented, on account of the flakes of coagulated fibrin which fill it.

The most rational treatment, therefore, if we get to the case early enough, is to irrigate the wound freely with a solution of carbolic acid in water (1 in 20), or with a solution of perchloride of mercury (1 in 1,000), injected by means of a glass syringe, or the pattern of syringe devised for quittor. This injecting should be done thoroughly, and by that we mean that several syringefuls of the solution should be injected, the joint after each injection being manipulated so as to distribute the solution as far as possible over it. When this is done the opening in the sole may be plugged with a little perchloride of mercury, or, better still, with a little piece of tow saturated with a concentrated solution of perchloride of mercury or a solution of iodoform in alcohol and an antiseptic pad of tow or lint placed over all. The foot should then be bandaged and encased in a boot or sacking protective. The bandage should be removed daily and the antiseptic pad changed. At each visit the animal's condition must be carefully noted. So long as constitutional disturbance is slight, the foot appears comfortable, is free from marked heat and tenderness, and pawing movements are absent, and so long as the discharge on the pad appears non-purulent, free from marked odour, and small in quantity, then this dressing may be persisted in.

This treatment of open joint, preventive as it is of arthritis, is also indicated in the case of open navicular bursa. In several instances we have practised this treatment for the dressing of wounds implicating the bursæ of tendons and the capsules of joints. It is also spoken of favourably by Mr. C.H. Flynn in the *American Veterinary Review* for June, 1888, whose treatment is as follows: 'Place the patient in a clean, well-ventilated, and drained stable. Have all the litter removed, and insist on the stall being kept clean. Either place the animal in slings, or tie the head so as to prevent lying down. Clip the hair and cleanse the parts well. He prefers the corrosive sublimate solution (1 in 1,000). Should the wound be of two or more days' standing, inject the joint with the corrosive sublimate solution. Now dry the parts with a clean towel and sprinkle the wound with iodoform. Over this place a thick layer of absorbent cotton-wool, filled with iodoform, bandage securely, and keep the patient on a moderate diet, preserving the utmost quietude possible. Should the bandage remain in position and the animal free from pain, leave the bandage and dressing in place from five days to a week. Then change it, and should the discharge be little, do not disturb it, but renew the iodoform and cotton dressing, leaving it on for another week.'

Other treatments for the same condition are practised, in which the wound is dusted with powdered iodoform, with potassium permanganate, or with corrosive sublimate, or where the wound, instead of being dusted, has the corrosive sublimate applied in the form of a plug. In each case the preliminary irrigation with the corrosive sublimate solution is dispensed with. This, however, should on no account be omitted. In our opinion it constitutes the very essence of the rationality of the treatment.

(b) Curative.–It may happen, however, and often does, that this first injection of an antiseptic is unsuccessful in preventing organismal infection of the wound. In this case grave constitutional disturbance and other untoward symptoms such as we have already described quickly make their appearance.

The animal should now be placed in slings and preparations made for actively treating the wound with antiseptics. Whether we fail or not, we have the satisfaction of knowing that we have given to the patient the best and the only chance of recovery.

It should be remembered, however, and should be pointed out to the owner, that with purulent arthritis fully developed, with the grave constitutional changes it occasions, and with the ever-present danger of a general septic invasion of the blood-stream, that the human surgeon under such circumstances offers to his patient the alternatives of amputation or probable death. With us no such alternative is possible. It is either return the joint to some semblance of its former usefulness, or destroy the patient.

In this case we advise the injection of the original wound, and also such fistulous openings as may have formed, with the 1 in 1,000 sublimate solution. Also, in order to avoid the sometimes abortive attempts of the antiseptic pad, to maintain a condition of asepsis around the wound, we advise the continual soaking of the whole foot in a cold antiseptic bath. This may be either carbolic acid 1 in 20, or–what is less volatile, perhaps more effectual, and certainly more economical–perchloride of mercury 1 in 1,000.

It has been our good fortune, even when we have seen the foot almost detached from the limb by the devastating inroads of the pus, to see the suppurative process by this means gradually overcome, a reparative anchylosis set in, and the animal restored to good health and usefulness, if not to soundness.

Once the suppurative process is checked and anchylosis commences, it is good treatment to smartly blister the whole of the region of the coronet, the pastern, and the wound itself with a mixed blister of cantharides and biniodide of mercury, repeated at intervals of a fortnight. This prevents to some extent further infection of the wound, and assists also in promoting the changes that tend to anchylosis.

(d) ANCHYLOSIS.

The word anchylosis signifies the stiffening of a joint. When one has read the serious changes occurring within the joint in the more serious forms of arthritis, it is easy to understand how it comes about. In suppurative arthritis, for instance, we have the synovial membrane destroyed, the articular cartilages partly or wholly obliterated, and the former boundaries of the joint entirely lost. If the animal lives, nature is bound to make repair of a sort. The synovial membrane and the articular cartilages utterly destroyed, as we have described, cannot again be replaced. Nature can only build again from such materials as are left to her. In this case the material is bone.

It must be remembered, however, that often the bone has been so diseased that spots of necrosis or caries within it are bound to remain unless moved by operative interference. Such diseased portions, when dealing with the foot, are beyond reach of the surgeon's knife, and we have no alternative but to allow them to remain. We get, therefore, in many cases, a condition of rarefactive ostitis occurring side by side with a slowly progressive caries within the bone, while outside is occurring an osteoplastic periostitis. The concurrence of these conditions leads in time to great increase in size of the parts, together with increasing anchylosis and deformity.

C. NAVICULAR DISEASE.

Definition.–Chronic inflammatory changes occurring in connection with the navicular bursa, affecting variously the bursa itself, the perforans tendon, or the navicular bone, and characterized by changes in the form of the hoof and persisting lameness. The disease is commonly noticed in thoroughbreds or in horses of the lighter breeds, and is but seldom observed in heavy cart animals. Usually it is met with in one or both fore-feet. Although of extremely rare occurrence, it has been noticed in the hind.

History.–To English veterinarians appears to belong the credit of discovering navicular disease. As early as 1752 we find one, Jeremiah Bridges, in 'No Foot, No Horse,' drawing attention to 'coffin-joint lameness,' and advocating for its treatment setoning of the frog. It appears, too, that Moorcroft, prior to his departure for India in 1808, was acquainted with what was then known as coffin-joint[A] lameness, having drawn attention to it in 1804 in a letter to Sir Edward Codrington.[B] In 1819 Moorcroft made it even plainer still that he was fully acquainted with what we now know as navicular disease. This we learn from a letter written by him to Sewell, in which he laid claim to being the originator of neurectomy. In this letter he says:

[Footnote A: The coffin-joint at this time included the navicular bursa.]

[Footnote B: Percival's 'Hippopathology,' vol. iv., p. 132.]

'On dissecting feet affected with these lamenesses, the flexor tendon was now and then observed to have been broken, partially or entirely, but more commonly to have been bruised and inflamed in its course under the navicular or shuttle bone, or at its insertion into the bone of the foot. Sometimes, although seldom, the navicular bone itself has been found to have been fractured; at others its surface has been deprived of its usual coating, and studded with projecting points or ridges of new growth, or exhibiting superficial excavations more or less extensive.'[A]

[Footnote A: *Ibid.*]

Pathology and Point of Commencement of the Disease.–The exact position in which the diseased process starts has for a long time been a subject of discussion, and even now it is doubtful whether the point has been definitely settled. To mention but a few among many: We find Mr. Broad, of Bath, strenuously insisting on the fact that the disease commences in the interior of the navicular bone. Just as strenuously we find the editor of the journal in which the matter is being discussed, the late Mr. Fleming, asserting that the disease commences in the bursa.[A] Others, too, hold that the disease commences primarily in the tendon. Wedded to this view was the discoverer, Mr. Turner, of Croydon; while Percival commits himself to the statement that it is either the central ridge or the postero-inferior surface of the navicular bone, or the opposed concavity in the perforans tendon, that shows the earliest signs of the disease. The observations made by Dr. Brauell, the first Continental writer to fully describe the disease, led him to the statement that neither the bone nor the bursa was the *invariable* starting-point of the trouble, but that usually it commenced in inflammation of the bursa itself.

[Footnote A: Percival's 'Hippopathology,' vol. iv., p. 132.]

Without, therefore, committing ourselves to an expression of opinion as to the precise starting-point of the affection, we shall describe the pathological changes occurring in navicular disease as noted in (1) the bursa, (2) the cartilage, (3) the tendon, and (4) the bone.

1. *Changes in the Bursa.*–Upon the internal surface of the bursal membrane is first noticed a slight inflammatory hyperæmia, accompanied by more or less swelling and tumefaction, owing to its infiltration with inflammatory exudate. The portion covering the hyaline cartilage of the navicular bone has lost its peculiar pearl-blue shimmer, and become a dirty yellow.

Remembering that the bursal membrane is a synovia-secreting one, and bearing in mind what happens in ordinary synovitis and arthritis (with which, of course, this may be very closely compared), we shall first expect changes in the bursal contents. It is highly probable, though difficult of proof, that in the very early stages the chronic inflammatory stimulus has the effect of increasing the flow of synovia. In every case, however, where it can with any certainty be said that navicular disease exists, it is too late to meet with this condition. The disease has then progressed until destruction of the secreting layer of the bursal membrane has been seriously interfered with, and in this case we find a distinct deficiency in the quantity of synovia in the bursa.

In advanced cases it is even found that the bursa is *absolutely dry*.

2. *Changes in the Cartilage*.–Directly that portion of the bursal membrane covering the cartilage is the subject of inflammatory change, the cartilage itself, by reason of its low vitality, soon suffers.

Under a process, which we may term 'dry ulcerative,' the cartilage covering the ridge on the lower surface of the bone commences to become eroded, and in appearance has been likened, both by English and Continental writers, to a piece of wood that has been worm-eaten (see Fig. 161).

'At this stage, or much earlier'–we are quoting Colonel Smith, A.V.D.–'may be found calcareous deposits in the fibro-cartilage and the bone. They are scattered like fine sand here and there, generally across the inferior half of the face of the bone; they are sometimes numerous, frequently scanty, occasionally entirely absent. The amount of calcareous degeneration depends upon the lesions present. If much destruction of bone exists, there will be but few calcareous deposits; whilst if there are many calcareous deposits, there may be but slight ulceration of bone tissue, and perhaps none at all. In fact, I have held the opinion, and see no reason to modify it, that calcareous deposits are safeguards against caries.'[A]

[Footnote A: *Journal of Comparative Pathology and Therapeutics*, vol. vi., p. 195.]

3. *Changes in the Tendon*.–The effect of these calcareous deposits on the under surface of the bone is to produce a certain amount of roughness. Seeing that with every movement of the foot the perforans tendon is called upon to glide over this surface, it is clear that a secondary effect must be that of inducing erosion and destruction of the tendon. The point at which this usually commences is at the bottom of the depression that accommodates the ridge on the bone. With erosion of the cartilage and of the tendon at points exactly opposite each other, we have two surfaces come together that are prone to readily unite, and fibrous tissue adhesions often take place between the bone and the tendon. In some measure this accounts for the torn and ragged ap-

pearance of the tendon. Adhesions take place, and, under some small strain, are broken down. This may happen more than once or twice, and with each breaking of the adhesion between the bone and tendon, fibres from the latter are lacerated and torn from their place (see Fig. 162).

4. *Changes in the Bone.*–The changes occurring in the bone are essentially those of a rarefactive ostitis. These changes are described by many writers, and, whether originating primarily in the bone or not, it seems certain that extensive changes may have occurred within the bone, with but little or nothing to be noted on its outer surface. It would seem that the first change is one of congestion of the vessels of the bone's cancellous tissue. With the cause, whatever it may be, in constant operation, the congestion persists until a low type of inflammation is set up, interfering, not only with the flow of synovia in the adjoining bursa, but with the nutrition of the bone itself. As the disease progresses, there is softening and enlarging of the cancellated tissue towards the centre of the bone. The cells break up, and absorption takes place. This goes on until a large portion of the interior of the bone is in a state of dry necrosis, with, in many cases, but slight signs of mischief on the exterior of the bone.

In other cases, however, the changes in the interior of the bone are accompanied by well-marked lesions on its gliding or postero-inferior surface, and by evidences of an osteoplastic periostitis along its edges.

That an osteoplastic periostitis has been in existence is witnessed by the appearance along the edges of the bone of numerous outgrowths of bone, termed osteophytes (see Fig. 163).

The interosseous and postero-lateral ligaments of the articulation often participate in the inflammatory changes, and in many cases become completely ossified. The true articulatory surface of the bone, that articulating with the os pedis and with the os coronæ, is never affected.

Causes.–In enumerating the causes of navicular disease, we shall follow the example of Colonel Smith and classify them under certain headings–namely,

(1) *Hereditary Predisposition*; (2) *Compression*; (3) *Concussion*; (4) *A Weak Navicular Bone*; (5) *A Defective or Irregular Blood-supply to the Bone*; and (6) *Senile Decay*.

1. *Hereditary Predisposition.*–That navicular disease is hereditary is a fact that has for a long time been insisted on, and has come to be so generally admitted that we do not intend to dwell on it here. As we have said before, it is found in the lighter breeds of horses (and, according to Zundel, especially in the English breeds), and is there seen to be frequently transmitted from parent to offspring.

2. *Compression.*–By this is meant the compression of the navicular bone between the os pedis and the os coronæ in front, and the perforans tendon behind.

In order to appreciate this explanation of the causation of navicular disease at its true value, it will be well to consider briefly the physiology of the parts in question.

The navicular bone is what we may term a complement of the os pedis. It exists, in fact, simply in order that the os coronæ may have a sufficiently large articulatory surface to play upon. One wonders at first that Nature did not arrive at this by originally placing a larger bone below. Colonel Smith explains this by suggesting that this would in all probability have meant its fracture. In progression the hind part of the foot comes to the ground first, and upon the hinder portion of the articulation would fall the first effects of concussion, together with the greater part of the body-weight. A yielding joint was in this position necessary, and that formed by the navicular bone fills all requirements.

In this connection one next considers the part played by the front limbs during progression. As Zundel expresses it, they are columns of support rather than of impulsion, and, as the body-weight is thrown forward by the hind-limbs, it is the duty of the fore-limbs to receive it. The shock or concussion of the body-weight thus thrown forwards is first received by the muscles uniting the limb to the trunk, and a great part of it there minimized by their sling-like attachment. It is further absorbed by the shoulder-joint, and from there passed on to the almost vertical bony column represented by the radius and ulna, the knee, and the metacarpus. On reaching the first phalanx, a portion of the remaining force is passed on to the front of the phalanges and loses itself in front of the hoof, while the other portion is transmitted to the flexor tendons, finally to the perforans, and to the posterior parts of the foot. During progression, therefore, the navicular bone is constantly pushed downwards and backwards by the bony column, and is just as constantly pushed forwards and upwards by the resistance of the perforans tendon. This means, of course, that the navicular bone is more or less constantly subject to compression, and constant pressure, as we know full well, is a pretty sure factor in bringing about malnutrition of the parts, with atrophy or chronic inflammatory changes as an end result.

Even with the limb at rest the pressure on both sides of the navicular bone is still constant. The only circumstances under which we can conceive of it being entirely absent, in fact, are when the tension on the tendon is relaxed, and the body-weight altogether removed by the animal adopting the recumbent position.

The compression theory as to the causation of navicular disease was, we believe, first originated by Colonel Smith. He, at any rate, has laid much stress on it in his writings. If we accept it, and we see every reason that we should, then we must, with the author, admit the possibility of navicular disease arising from long standing in one position.

3. *Concussion.*–This we are bound to admit as a cause, and in so doing partly explain the comparative, almost total, immunity of the hind-feet from the disease. The fore-limbs, as we have already pointed out, are little more than props of support, and the force of the propelled body-weight is transmitted largely down their almost vertical lines, to end largely in concussion in the foot. With the hind-limbs matters are different. 'These,' as Percival explains it, 'have their bones obliquely placed, so as to constitute, one with the other,

so many obtuse angles, to the end, that by forming powerful levers, and affording every advantage for action to the muscles attached to them, they may be fitted for the purpose of propulsion of the body onward.'

The effect of these several obtuse-angled joints in the limb is to absorb the greater part of the force exerted by the body-weight before it reaches the foot. When with this we take the facts that the fore-limbs have to carry the head and neck, and that they have to bear this added weight, plus a propelling force from behind, we see why it is that they should be so subject to the disease, and the hind-limbs so exempt.

As pointing out the part that concussion plays in its causation, we may mention that navicular disease is a disease of the middle-aged and the worked animal. It is interesting to note, too, that it occurs in animals with well developed frogs–in feet in which frog-pressure with the ground is most marked. This at first sight appears to flatly contradict what we have said with regard to frog-pressure in other portions of this work. With this, however, must be reckoned other predisposing causes. In this case it is not to frog-pressure alone we must look, but to the condition of the frog itself, and that of the neighbouring parts. It is when we have a frog which, though well developed and apparently satisfying all demands as to size and build, is at the same time composed of a hard, dry, and non-yielding horn that we must look for trouble.

The foot predisposed to navicular disease is the strong, round, short-toed or clubby foot, open at the heels, with a sound frog jutting prominently out between them. Here is a frog exposed to all the pressure that might be desired for it, bounded at its sides by heels thick and strong, and indisposed to yield, and itself liable, from its very exposure, to become, in the warm stable, hard and dry, and incompressible' (Percival).

Here, instead of acting, as normally it should, as a resilient body, and an aid to the absorption of concussion, it seems rather to play the part of a foreign body, and to bring concussion about. Seeing, then, that the navicular bursa is in very near contact with it, it is conceivable that this joint-like apparatus should suffer, and the pedal articulation be left unaffected, the more so when we take into consideration the compression theory just described.

4. *A Weak Navicular Bone.*–When the disease commences first in the bone–and there is no denying the fact that sometimes, although not invariably, it does–it may be explained by attributing to the structure of the bone an abnormal weakness in build.

The navicular bone consists normally of compact and cancellated tissue arranged in certain proportions, the compact tissue without, and the cancellated within. These proportions can only be judged of by the examinations of sections of the bone, and when it is found in any case that the cancellated tissue bulks more largely in the formation of the bone than normally it should, we have what we may term a weak navicular bone. In this connection Colonel Smith says: 'Though it is far from present in every case of the disease, still I consider it a factor of great importance.'

5. *A Defective or Irregular Blood-supply to the Bone.*–This, Colonel Smith considers, is brought about by excessive and irregular work, and by the opposite condition–rest. The author points out that the bloodvessels passing to and from the navicular bone run in the substance of the interosseous ligaments, or in such proximity to them that it is conceivable that under certain circumstances mechanical interference may occur to the navicular circulation. He further points out a fact that is, of course, well known to every veterinarian, that in periods of work the circulation of the foot is hurried, and that in rest there is always a tendency to congestion; and he says in conclusion: 'I cannot help thinking that irregularities in the blood-supply in a naturally weak bone must be a factor of some importance, especially when the kind of work the horse is performing is a series of vigorous efforts followed by rest.'

6. *Senile Decay.*–With approaching age the various tissues lose their vigour, and are prone to disease. The navicular bone and surrounding structures are

not exempt. With the other and more active causes we have described acting at the same time it is not surprising that navicular disease is seen as a result.

In conclusion, it is well, perhaps, to say that, no matter to which particular theory of causation we may lean, we should make up our minds to consider them as a whole. While one cause may be exciting, the other may be predisposing, and the two must act together before evil results are noticed. It may be that even more than two are concerned in bringing on the disease, and to each the careful veterinarian will give due consideration.

Symptoms and Diagnosis.–In the early stages of navicular disease the symptoms are obscure. Pointing of the affected limb is the first evidence the animal gives. This, however, more often than not, goes unnoticed, and the first symptom usually observed by the owner or attendant is the lameness. Even this is such as to at first occasion no alarm, being intermittent and slight, and only very gradually becoming marked. In a few cases, however, lameness will come on suddenly, and is excessive from the commencement. It is the lameness, slow in its onset, intermittent in its character, and gradual in its progress, however, that is ordinarily characteristic of navicular disease.

The animal is taken out from the stable sound, with just a vague suspicion, perhaps, that he moved a bit stiffly. While out he is thought by his driver or rider to be going feelingly with one foot or with both. Even this is not marked, and the driver has some difficulty in assuring himself whether or no he really observed it, or whether it was but imagination.

On the return home the limb is examined, and nothing abnormal is to be found. The leg is of its normal appearance, and neither heat nor tenderness is to be observed in it or in the foot. On the following day the animal again is sound, and the lameness of the previous day is put down to a slight strain or something equally simple. The patient is then, perhaps, rested for a day or two. When next he is worked he again moves out from the stable sound, but again during the going gives the driver the unpleasant impression that something is amiss; and so the case goes on. One day the owner fears the animal is becoming seriously enough affected to warrant him in calling in his veterinary surgeon; the next he is confidently assuring himself that nothing is wrong.

Perhaps the animal is now rested for a week or two, or even for a month or two, hoping that this will put him sound. Immediately on commencing work, however, the same symptoms as before assert themselves, and the veterinary surgeon is called in.

With a history such as we have given the veterinarian's suspicions are aroused. He has the animal trotted, and may notice at this stage that there is an inclination to go on the toes, that the lame limb or limbs are not put forward freely, and that progression is stilty and uncertain; it is such, in fact, as to at once suggest the possibility of corns being present.

In some cases there is just the suspicion of a limp with one limb, and this only at intervals during the trot. At one moment the veterinarian is positive that he sees the animal going lame; at another he is just as confident he sees him coming towards him sound.

Nothing is found in the limb–neither heat, tenderness, nor swelling. There is nothing in the gait (either a limited movement of the radius, or a circular sweep with the leg) to indicate shoulder or other lameness, and the veterinary surgeon, by eliminative evidence, is bound to conclude that the trouble is in the foot.

The foot is then examined–pared, percussed, pinched, and in other ways manipulated–but nothing further is forthcoming. In such a case the veterinary surgeon is wise to declare the abortive result of his examination, to hint darkly of his suspicions, and to suggest a second examination at some future date. It may be that two, three, four, or even more, such examinations are necessary before he can justly pronounce a positive verdict.

Later he is enabled to do this by an increase in the severity of the symptoms, and by the changes that take place in the form of the foot. The lameness is now more marked, and the 'pointing' in the stable more frequent. With regard to the latter symptom, it has been seriously discussed whether the horse with navicular disease points with the heel elevated or with it pressed to the ground. In either case, of course, the limb is advanced; but while some hold that the phalangeal articulations are flexed and the heel slightly raised, in order to relieve the pressure of the perforans tendon on the affected area, and so obtain ease, there are others who hold that the heel is pressed firmly to the ground in order to deaden the pain. It may be, and most probably is, that both are right; but, in our opinion, there is no doubt whatever that pointing with the heel elevated is by far the most common.

The lameness is now excessive, and is especially noticeable when the animal is put to work on a rough or on a hard ground. Even now, however, heat of the foot or tenderness is so slight as to be out of all proportion to the alteration in gait.

With the case thus far advanced, evidence of pain may be obtained by pressing with the thumb in the hollow of the heel. Evidence of pain may also be obtained by using the farrier's pincers on the frog. These methods, however, are never wholly satisfactory, as a horse with the soundest of feet will sometimes flinch under these manipulations.

Extreme and forcible flexion of the corono-pedal articulation also sometimes gives evidence of tenderness. In this case the foot is held up, the animal's metacarpus resting on the operator's knee, and the toe of the hoof pushed downwards with some degree of force.

The same movement of the joint is given by causing the animal to put full weight upon the diseased limb, a small wedge of wood being first placed under the toe. In this manner the pressure of the perforans tendon upon the bursa is greatly increased, and the animal is caused to show symptoms of distress.

The lameness may also be increased, and diagnosis helped, by paring the heels, so as to leave the frog prominent and take the whole of the body-weight. The same end is also obtained by applying a bar shoe. This was originally pointed out by Brauell, and is quoted by Zundel and by Möller.

The changes in the form of the hoof may now be noticed. These are largely dependent on the fact that more or less constantly the patient saves the heel. The horn of the walls in this region, and the horn of the frog, is thereby put out of action and induced to atrophy. The hoof gradually assumes a more upright shape, and the heels contract. We thus get a hoof which is visibly narrowed from side to side, with a frog that is atrophied and often thrushy, and with a sole that is abnormally concave, hard, and affected with corns.

When occurring in the hind-feet–a condition that is rare, but which has been noticed by Loiset, and quoted by Zundel–the animal is stiff behind, walks on his toes, and gives one the impression that he is suffering from some affection in the region of the loins.

One such case is reported by an English veterinary surgeon, and we quote it here:

'A gray gelding, and a capital hunter, the property of a gentleman in this neighbourhood, became lame in the near fore-foot after the hunting season of 1859. The lameness was believed to be due to navicular disease. The operation of neurectomy was ultimately had recourse to. The horse subsequently did his work as well as ever, and was ridden to hounds regularly till the end of the year 1861, when he went lame of the off fore-foot. From this date he also showed very peculiar action behind, and was at times lame of both hind-limbs without any apparent cause.

'In the year 1862, from the groom's indiscreet use of physic, superpurgation was brought on which caused the animal's death. On a post-mortem examination being made, the horse was found to have *navicular disease of all four feet.* It is worthy of note that this horse had always "extravagant" action behind, but was a remarkably quick and good jumper.'[A]

[Footnote A: F. Blakeway, M.R.C.V.S., *Veterinarian*, vol. ii., p. 21.]

Differential Diagnosis.–Navicular disease may be mistaken for ordinary contracted foot. It will be remembered, however, that in the early stages of navicular disease contraction is absent, and that it is only when the disease in the bursa is of long standing that contraction comes on. With ordinary contracted foot, too, careful paring and suitable shoeing soon sees a diminution in the degree of lameness, and a return to the normal in shape (see Treatment of Contracted Foot, p. 125). With navicular disease, however, such shoeing as is beneficial in the treatment of contracted foot (notably the various methods of giving to the frog counter-pressure with ground) soon brings on an aggravation of the lameness.

It is, perhaps, even more likely to be confounded with contraction when we have with the contraction a state of atrophy and thrush of the frog. With a frog in this condition pressure will give rise to pain, and navicular disease be erroneously judged to be present. In such a case we must rely wholly upon either extreme flexion or extreme extension of the joint to guide us, when, if contraction *only* is the offending condition, no symptom of pain will be shown.

Navicular disease may also be confused with rheumatic affections, with sprain of the posterior ligaments of the first interphalangeal articulation, and with sesamoid lameness. Mistakes are sometimes made, too, especially with a hasty observer, in confounding it with shoulder lameness.

In rheumatism the constant changing of the seat of pain, the sometimes elevated temperature, and the appearance of symptoms of heat, tenderness, and swelling in the affected area should guide one to a right conclusion.

In sprain of the posterior ligaments of the coronet and in sesamoid lameness, nothing but a careful examination and manipulation of the parts will ward off error, for in each of these cases there is 'pointing' and resting of the limb, and considerable disinclination to put weight firmly upon it. If at the same time manipulation gives distinct evidence of pain, all doubt may be set at rest.

Roughly speaking, sesamoid lameness is a condition of the gliding surface of the sesamoids, and the face of the tendon playing over them, similar to that found in navicular disease. All symptoms of pointing, the constant maintaining of the limb in a state of flexion, and a feeling manner of progression are again all present. It is plain from this that in all cases where an animal with a gait at all suggestive of navicular disease is brought for our examination, the manipulation of the limb should be thorough. The character of the lameness is almost sure to deceive us; and it is not until we are able to obtain local symptoms pointing to the one or the other of the conditions we have enumerated that a decisive opinion may be given. In sesamoid lameness the local symptoms are those of heat and pain in the fetlock on palpation, and a swelling of the affected parts, such swelling being at first slight, yielding, and barely distinguishable, and afterwards larger, bony and hard, and more marked. Later still there is distinct evidence of 'knuckling' over at the fetlock and inability to fully flex it.

In cases of shoulder lameness the gait alone should be sufficient to render liability of error small, for with nearly every case there is a manifest inability to 'get the limb forward', and this is best seen at a side view when the animal is trotting past the observer. When trotting towards one, there is a further and unmistakable symptom common to most shoulder lamenesses that serves to distinguish it at once, and that is the peculiar 'sweeping' outwards with the affected limb.

Lastly, with either of the conditions we have just mentioned, it is the exception to get contracted foot follow on. With navicular disease it sooner or later makes its appearance.

Prognosis.–The prognosis of navicular disease (once diagnosed with certainty) must almost of necessity be unfavourable. The facts that the disease has made serious progress before it is really noticeable, that the situation of the parts prohibits operative interference, and that the disease is one of a chronic and slowly progressive type, all point to an unfavourable termination.

Treatment.–We have seen from the pathology of this disease that it may commence either as a rarefactive ostitis, or as a synovitis and tenositis in connection with the bursa. With the former condition in existence, or when this and the synovitis has led to erosion of the cartilage, treatment is probably of no avail, on account of the more chronic nature of these two conditions. When, however, the condition is simply that of synovitis or tenositis, a more or less acute condition, we may assume that suitable treatment and a long rest will bring about resolution.

The first indications in treatment are those of what we may term 'nursing' the foot. It should have sufficient rest, should be placed so as to minimize as far as possible compression of the parts, and should have its posterior half treated so as to render it softer and less liable to concussion.

The period of rest required cannot be satisfactorily advised, and the practitioner is wise who makes it a long one. Best should be advised, in fact, long after symptoms of lameness have disappeared and recovery is judged to have taken place.

Compression of the parts may be somewhat minimized, if the animal be kept in the stable, by allowing the floor upon which the front-feet are to stand to be slightly sloping from behind forwards. The same effect, though not so marked, is obtained by removing the shoes, and considerably lowering the wall at the toe, while allowing that of the heels to remain. It may here be remarked that it is a good practice to allow the shoes to remain on, and this even when the animal is at grass. They should, however, be frequently removed, and the foot trimmed as we have directed.

With the foot thus trimmed so as to most suitably adjust the angles of the articulations, it should next be thoroughly pared and rasped in its posterior half, so as to render the horn of the sole and the frog and the horn of the quarters as thin as possible. The heels, however, should not be excessively lowered, *if at all.* We now have the foot in a soft condition, and easily expanded. It should, if possible, be kept so; and this may be done either by the use of poultices, by tepid baths, or by standing the animal upon a bedding that may easily be kept constantly damp. Such materials as tan, peat moss, or sawdust, are either of them suitable.

All this, of course, calls for keeping the animal in the stable. It is far better, however, more especially if a piece of marshy land is at hand, to turn him out in that. A moderate amount of exercise is beneficial rather than not, and the feet are thus constantly kept damp without trouble to the attendants.

The second indication in the treatment is that of applying a counter-irritant as near to the diseased parts as possible. Regarding its efficacy we must confess to being somewhat sceptical. The treatment has been constantly practised and advised, however, and we feel bound to give it mention here. A smart blister may, therefore, be applied to the whole of the coronet, and need not be prevented from running into the hollow of the heel.

Instead of blistering the coronet (or in conjunction with that treatment), the counter-irritant may be applied by passing a seton through the plantar cushion or fibro-fatty frog. Setoning the frog appears to have been introduced by Sewell. In many cases great benefit is claimed to have been derived from it, especially by English veterinarians of Sewell's time, and by others on the Continent. Percival, however, was not an advocate for it, and, at the present day, it is a practice which appears to have dropped out of use altogether.

To perform this operation a seton needle of a curved pattern is needed (see Fig. 164). This is threaded with a piece of stout tape dressed with a cantharides, hellebore, or other blistering ointment, and then passed in at the hollow of the heel, emerging at the point of the frog. The course the needle should take will be understood from a reference to Fig. 165.

The seton may be passed with the horse in the standing position. Previously the point of the frog should be thinned, and the animal should be twitched. After-treatment consists simply in moving the seton daily, and dressing it occasionally with any stimulating ointment, or with turpentine.

If, in spite of these treatments, the disease persists, then nothing remains but neurectomy.

D. DISLOCATIONS.

The firm and rigid manner in which the bones of the pedal articulation are held together renders dislocation of this joint an exceedingly rare occurrence, and then it is only liable to happen under the operation of great force. In the literature to our hand we have only been successful in discovering one reported instance, and, strange to say, in this, a well-marked case, the cause was altogether obscure. We quote the case at the end of this section.

A partial dislocation of this articulation is the condition met with in 'Buttress Foot.' In this case the fracture of the pyramidal process, and the consequent lengthening of the tendon of the extensor pedis, allows the os coronæ to occupy upon the articulatory surface of the os pedis a more backward position than normally it should.

It is quite probable, too, that slight lesions of the other restraining ligaments and tendons of the articulation may bring about a similar though less marked condition. We may be quite sure of this–that whenever such lesions (as, for example, sprain and partial rupture of the lateral ligaments) do occur, and the normal position of the opposing bones is changed, if only slightly, that great pain and excessive lameness must be the result, and this with but little to show in the foot. Many of our cases of obscure foot lameness might, if capable of demonstration, turn out to be cases of sprain and partial dislocation of the pedal articulation.

Recorded Case.–'The animal, a trooper of the 8th Hussars, was found on the morning of April 17 unable to bear any weight on the limb (the near hind). Cause not known–the heel-rope I thought at first; but on investigation I found the heel-rope had been on the other leg.

Diagnosis.–Dislocation of the left os coronæ from the articulating surface of the os pedis in a backward direction.

'Every devisable means were unsuccessful in reducing the limb to its natural position. The horse was thrown, and a strong rope, with four men pulling at it, was fastened round the hoof, whilst I put my knee to the back of the pastern, using all possible force, with one hand to the foot and the other to the fetlock, but all to no purpose. Next day other means were tried. First by throwing the horse and placing him on his belly, with the fore-legs stretched out forwards, and the hind-legs backwards. This I did so as to get the injured limb placed as nearly flat on the ground as possible, with its anterior aspect downwards. Then a very heavy man, with his boots off, was made to jump on the back of the pastern, where the prominence showed most; and afterwards, when these means failed, a strong piece of wood, well covered with leather, was placed (where the hollow of the heel ought to have been) on the most prominent part, and hit several times with a heavy hammer; but all efforts were futile.

'*Prognosis.*–Unfavourable. During the latter operations I had a very strong pressure applied to the hoof, and the horse firmly fastened in every way, and it appeared as though no amount of force would ever reduce the dislocation.

'*Tautological.*–The case was destroyed on April 30, being of no further use to the service.

'*Post-mortem.*–The os coronæ was found to have slipped out of the articulating cavity of the os pedis, backwards and past the lateral ligaments. These last-named structures prevented the bone being forced forward into its proper position, being firmly locked over the lateral prominences. The capsular ligament was considerably lacerated and inflamed, causing slight effusion and swelling about the region of the coronet.'[A]

[Footnote A: T. Flintoff, A.V.D., *Veterinary Journal*, vol. xix., p. 74.]

Treatment.–After the forcible means of reduction related by Mr. Flintoff, we may add that when they are successful, they should be followed by suitable bandaging of the parts, and rest. The first is effected by applying plaster of Paris and linen, and the second by having the animal put in slings.

INDEX

THE END